Secrets Of Having Strong Bone

In The Body.

I0505343

Olatundun Solomon

olatundunsolomon@gmail.com

Olatundun Solomon has distinction in the program Diploma in Nursing and Patient Care.

He has distinction in the program Diploma in Human Nutrition.

He has Honor code certificate from Karolinska Institutet in edx. The course is KIBEHMEDx:

Behavioral Medicine: A Key to Better Health.

From the University of Queensland in edx he has the certificate BIOIMG101x: Introduction to Biomedical Imaging.

From Harvard University in edx he has the certificate HSPH-HMS214x: Fundamentals of Clinical Trials.

From Harvard University he also has the certificate PH201x: Health and Society. From the University of Texas System in edx he has the certificate 4.01x: Take Your Medicine - The Impact of Drug Development.

The Bone:

The bone is very important in the human body. It is a crucial organ that is rigid. It makes up the skeletal system of the body. It is a structure that helps in the protection of tissues and organs in the body. The heart is protected, the lungs are protected and other tissues in the body. Bone is located in the head, neck,

arms,

hands,

chest,

back,

thigh,

legs,

feet and different parts of the

body.

Inside the bone is the marrow.

From the bone marrow, white

blood cells and red blood cells

are produced. Red blood cells helps in the transportation of oxygen in the body. White blood cells helps to fight against infections. In the body the femur located in the thigh in the lower limb is a long bone. The bones in the wrist and ankle are short bones. Flat bone is the sternum located in the chest. The bone together with ligaments, tendons and muscles helps the body to move from

one place to the other. The

bone helps in the storing of

minerals such as calcium,

magnesium and phosphorous.

Osseous tissue of the body

which is bone tissue is dense

connective tissue. This makes

the bone to be strong.

Osteoblasts and also osteocytes

bone cells helps the body to

form bone growth and development. That is, the mineralize bone occurs. And osteoclast makes bone resorption to occur, this helps in regulating the calcium level of the bone. In order for the body to have normal bone density. Collagen known as ossein is protein that helps in the building up of the bone, by strengthening it.

Bone is divided into cortical bone and cancellous bone. Cortical bone is also known as compact bone. And cancellous bone is also known as spongy bone.

Cortical bone is the outer cortex layer of the bone while the spongy bone is the inner spongy part of the bone. There are some other tissues that are attached to the bone. These are blood vessels, nerves, cartilage, bone marrow, peristeum and endosteum.

1. Blood vessels: This makes blood to be transported to the bones in the body. This makes oxygen to get to different bones of the body. The oxygen is carried by the iron in the hemoglobin in the red blood cell. It is very important not to smoke, because this makes free

radicals to carry the oxygen.

This makes the bone not to be

nourished by oxygen. It will

then make the bone to be weak.

This makes the bone to be at

risk of fracture. This can make

the bone to be easily affected

by other diseases. When there

is injury that causes blood

vessels that supply a bone to

cut, it can lead to the death of

such a bone because of the lack

of nourishment of the blood to the bone. In the blood there are vitamins and minerals that makes the bone to be strong and healthy. When blood is not supplied to a particular bone due to the cut of blood vessels that supplied the bone. These minerals and vitamins will not be able to reach the bone to nourish it. This will cause malnourishment to the bone.

But when there is good supply of blood to the bones, this makes nutrients and oxygen to be transported to the bone for nourishment. This will make the bone to be mineralized normally, this will make the bone density to be increased and therefore the bone will be strong and healthy.

The arteries carry oxygenated blood to the bone for

nourishment. But the

pulmonary artery carry

deoxygenated blood to the

lungs. The veins carry

deoxygenated blood to the

lungs to be oxygenated. But the

pulmonary vein carry

oxygenated blood.

2. Nerves: The nerves helps in

the transmission of sensory

impulses to and from the bone.

This makes the bone to be able

to feel pain, heat, cold and touch. The basic unit of the nerve is neuron. There are motor neuron and sensory neuron. The motor neuron relay impulses from the brain to the spinal cord and from the spinal cord to the bone. Sensory neuron relay impulses from the bone to the spinal cord and from the spinal cord to the brain. When there is cut of the nerves that supply a particular

bone, it makes the bone not to

be noticed by the brain. This

will make sensation of the

particular bone to be lost. It is

therefore important to wear sit

belt in the car to prevent

accident that can lead to cut of

the nerve supply. It is good to

make the house to be free from

dirts scattered around. It is

good not to let knives to be

improperly placed in the house. This will prevent accident.

3. Cartilage: This is attached to the bone. It makes movement to be possible during stretching of the body. Elastic cartilage makes elasticity of the body to occur. The cartilage is usually attach to the bone some will eventually ossify in adult. When there is wear of the cartilage due to over use of the joints. It

makes pain to occur in that area

of the joint. For example, in the

case of arthritis. Food that are

good in lubricating the joints are

avocado,

soy bean,

sardine and vegetable oil.

Infection to the joint can be

prevented by eating antibiotic

food, such as curry powder,

ginger,

thyme and various spices.

4. Bone marrow: From the bone marrow, white blood cells (leukocytes), red blood cells (erythrocytes) and platelets (thrombocytes) are produced.

The White blood cells helps the body to fight against infections. The red blood cells helps in the carrying of oxygen to different parts of the body and the platelets helps in the clotting of blood (hemostasis) during hemorrhage (bleeding) after injury. It is very good to eat green vegetables because of the presence of folic acid. This helps in the production of blood in the bone marrow. This makes the bone to be well nourished. This will make the bone strong and healthy.

5. Peristeum: This covers the outer part of the bone.

6. Endosteum: This covers the inner part of the cortex of the bone.

The bone is divided in to different groups, these are:

1. Long bones

2. Short bones

3.Flat bones

4. Irregular bones

5. Sesamoid bones and

6. Sutural bones.

1. Long bones are located in the arm. This is the humerus. Long bone is also located in the thigh. This is the femur.

2. Short bones: These are located in the wrist. This are the carpal bones. They are also found in the ankles. This are tarsal bones.

3. Flat bones: These are bones that are flat. Example is the sternum, it is located in the chest.

4. Irregular bones: Examples are located in the skull, which are sphenoid and ethmoid bones.

5. Sesamoid bones: Example of this bone is located in the knee. This is called the knee cap(patella).

6. Sutural bones: These bones are located in the skull.

Function Of The Bone.

1. The bone is used for hearing. The three ossicles which are bones located in the middle ear helps in hearing.

2. From the bone marrow white blood cells(leukocytes), red blood cells(erythrocytes) and platelets(thrombocytes) are produced. When the bone cells are well produced, it prevent anemia. Anemia is when the blood level of the body is below

normal. This can occur when there is bone marrow disease. It can also occur due to malnutrition. When fruits, green vegetables, beans, fish, egg, beef, chicken, turkey, wheat, yam, potato, rice are not eaten moderately. It is important to eat balance diet. This helps to prevent anemia. It is good to be free from mosquito bite. This prevent suck of blood from mosquito. Suck of blood from mosquito can cause anemia. It is good to use mosquito net, in order to prevent mosquito bite.

3. The collagen of the bone, helps in bone elasticity. It strengthens the bone. The collagen is protein. It is good to eat protein food, such as fish,

beef,

egg,

beans,

chicken,

turkey and liver. This helps in
the formation of collagen. It is
good to eat balance diet.

4. There is attachment of
ligaments, tendons, skeletal
muscles and joints in the body.
This helps in the body
movement. There are
attachment of muscles in the

body to skeletons. This is called skeletal muscles. This muscles together with ligaments, tendons and joints helps in movement of the body. When there is tear of ligament, tendon or skeletal muscle, the area that is torn, movement will be difficult in that area, and it is painful. Moderate exercise is needed and not to over use the joints that can lead to the tear of tendon, cartilage or skeletal

muscle.

5. Bones helps in the storing of

minerals such as calsium,

phosphorus and magnesium. it

is good to eat food that has

these minerals, in order for the

bone to be mineralized and

there is no risk of fracture of the

bone. This can be found in

green leafy vegetables.

6. Bones helps in regulating the acid and the base balance of the human body.

7. Bones gives structure and shape to the human body. It is good to prevent bone diseases, in order to prevent improper shape of the bone. This can be noticed in paget's disease of the bone. It is good to use drug prescription well in order to not cause adverse effects on the

bone of the body. It is good to drink clean water in order to prevent water borne diseases. It is good to have good body hygiene in order to prevent communicable diseases that can affect the bone negatively and the entire body.

8. The bones helps many structures to be protected, such as the heart, lungs and the brain. The heart is protected by the

ribs and sternum. The brain is

protected by the skull. The

lungs are protected by the

sternum and the ribs.

How To Have Strong And Healthy Bone.

1. Exercise: Exercise is physiotherapy where by bone density increases. This makes the bone to be healthy and strong. This prevent osteoporosis and osteomalacia. Osteoporosis is porosity that

occur to the bone. This makes

the bone to be very weak.

Osteomalacia means the bone is

soft. Physiotherapy can be done

through exercises to increase

the bone density. Exercise can

be done by jogging, walking,

swimming, stretching of the

body, by doing press up and by

doing yo yo. Exercise helps in

the prevention of obesity. This

makes ill health of the bone by

obesity to be prevented.

2. Vitamin K: This vitamin helps

in the increase of bone density.

Bone mineralization occur.

Example of food that has

vitamin K are green leafy

vegetables such as

spinach,

 cabbage,

broccoli and lettuce. Vegetable oil has vitamin K, also nuts, fruits such as berries, grapes and figs have vitamin K. Soya beans and liver also have vitamin K.

4. Vitamin C (Ascorbic acid) helps in the synthesis of collagen and also helps in the stimulation of procollagen. This keeps the bone strong and

healthy. Vitamins C is found in

citrus fruits such as lemon,

guava,

lime and orange. Other vitamin

C source are kiwifruits, broccoli,

raw bell pepper,

strawberry,

peach,

onion,

watermelon,

apple,

carrot,

avocado and cherry.

 Vitamin C is also in red and

green peppers,

tomatoes,

spinach,

peas,

potatoes,

cauliflower,

cabbage,

Brussels sprouts,

cantaloupe,

strawberries and kiwifruits.

Vitamin C act as cofactor in the hydroxylation of lysin and proline. It helps in collagen fibrils crosslinking. Osteoblast is formed as a result of alkaline phosphatase action that is stimulated as a result of vitamin

C presence. This makes the

bone to be mineralized.

Therefore the density of the

bone is increased. This makes

the bone to be strong.

5. Vitamin B12: Vitamin B12 is

found in fish,

turkey,

chicken,

goat meat and ram meat. With

the aid of vitamin B12

osteoblast works properly.

Vitamin B12 helps the

erythrocytes (red blood cells) to

mature. The osteoblast then

makes the bone to be

mineralized and the bone

density increases. Vitamin B12

is cofactor for example,

osteocalcin and alkaline

phosphatase. By the action of

vitamin B12 bone is formed due

to the metabolism of iron. Due

to the bone formation that occurred, osteoporosis is prevented. This makes the bone to be strong and in good health.

6. Vitamin E: Vitamin E has anti-inflammatory and also antioxidant action, and it go against free radicals that can cause bone cell damage. This therefore prevent demineralization of the bone. This makes the bone not to be

thin. This then prevent the bone from risk of fracture.

Sources of vitamin E are:

Peanuts,

soybean oil,

corn oil,

peanut oil,

chicken,

grape seed oil,

avocado,

cashew nuts,

spinach,

beef,

palm oil,

popcorn,

broccoli,

brown rice,

fish,

milk and

egg.

7. Magnesium, Calcium and Phosphorus: These minerals helps in the building up of bone cells, thereby increasing bone density. This makes the bone to be strong and healthy. Fruits that has magnesium, calcium and phosphorus are raspberry, pumpkins,

lettuce and squash. Food that

has magnesium are legumes,

nuts, and green vegetables.

Food that contain calcium are

sardines,

salmon,

cheese and

soybeans.

8. Prevent obesity: Bone good

health is high when obesity is

prevented. The use of vegetable

oil and not animal fat for

cooking is healthy to the bone.

Animal fat can cause obesity

which is not healthy for the

bone. It is therefore good to eat

moderately. When animal fat is

eaten, it can cause narrowing of

the arteries(atherosclerosis).

This can make small amount of

blood to flow to the bone,

thereby causing the bone to be

undernourished.

Undernourishment of the bone
makes the bone not to be
strong and healthy. It is
therefore, good to use
vegetable oil in food. Eating of
balance diet is good. Too much
eating of carbohydrates and
leaving protein, minerals,
vitamins and vegetable oil not
taken as food can cause obesity.
It is therefore good to eat
moderately. Obesity can be

treated by the use of

physiotherapy (exercise),

phytotherapy (use of plant food

such as cucumber,

lime,

lemon and

garden egg.

Cabbage and lettuce also helps,

because of high fiber) and the

use of sitotherapy(use of food

such as beans because of the fiber content).

9. Improve sleep: It is good to sleep well for good bone growth. Growth hormone is produced at night. It is good to sleep well at night for proper bone growth. When you sleep well it makes the bone to be strong.

10. It is good for pregnant women to eat healthy balance

diet. This makes the fetus in her uterus(womb) to be healthy and there is going to be formation of healthy bones in the fetus.

11. Vitamin A: It is important in the proper shaping of the bone. The bone cells osteoblast and osteoclasts has receptor for retinoic acid. This makes the bone to be in proper shape. This prevent abnormal bone shape.

Food that has vitamin A are

mangoes,

pawpaw,

oil palm fruits,

carrots,

cod liver oil,

milk,

pea,

egg,

tomatoes,

spinach,

bell pepper,

pumpkin,

fish,

squash,

sweet potato,

butternut,

liver of turkey,

liver of chicken and liver of beef.

12. Iron: This is mineral that it's activity is a cofactor for the synthesis of collagen bone matrix. This activity is done in enzyme.

12. Manganese: It helps as cofactor for many enzymes in the bone tissue. It also helps in mucopolysaccharides biosynthesis in the formation of bone matrix.

13. Copper: This helps in the formation of bone. Bone connective tissue becomes normal. The bone becomes well mineralized.

14. Zinc: Zinc act in osteoblast actions. Collagen is synthesized by it. Zinc also helps in the renewing of bone tissues. It also helps in the mineralization of the bone. Food that has zinc are turkey, chicken,

cereals,

pulses and beef.

15. Fluoride: This is needed by the bone. It prevent demineralization of the bone. Onion is food source for fluoride.

16. Vitamin D: This vitamin is gotten from the early morning sun. It makes the bone of the body to absorb calcium. Calcium can be reduced by too much

intake of caffeine and salt.

When there is vitamin D

deficiency the bone in the body

is at risk of fracture. Food that

as vitamin D are sardines,

salmon,

tuna,

liver,

egg,

mackerel,

lamb and hen.

17. Protein: Protein is food that

helps in bone growth and

development. Protein food are

fish,

egg,

milk,

liver,

beans,

pea nuts and beef.

18. Vegetables: When vegetables are eaten it increases the density of the bone. Vegetables are lettuce and cabbage.

Fracture:

Fracture occurs when the bone breaks. This can occur during accident. It can also occur after a very long walk and there is no rest, for example, microfracture.

Types Of Fracture:

There are different types of

fracture.

1. Transverse fracture

2. Open fracture

3. Closed fracture

4. Oblique fracture

5. Spiral fracture

6. Microfracture

1. Transverse fracture: This type
of fracture is the type that can
occur to the bone. And the bone
has fracture that is right angle
to the bone long axis. This can
easily occur when the bone is

weak. That is the bone density is low.

2. Open fracture: Open fracture is a type of fracture that is also called compound fracture. In this type of fracture, the wound that is formed after the trauma(injury) communicate with the fracture that occurred.

3. Closed fracture:

This type of fracture is the type that the bone is fractured and there is there skin that is still covering it. That is the bone is not seen outside of the body.

4. Oblique fracture: This is a type of fracture that occur to the bone that is diagonal to the bone long axis. That is the fracture occur obliquely to the bone long axis.

5. Spiral fracture: This is a type of fracture that the bone has twist form. That is the fracture is in spiral form.

6. Microfracture: This is fracture that occur, that can be investigated by the use of Xray or CT scan. This can occur after a very long distance walk without resting. It is good to have a lot of rest and eat food that can aid bone development.

In the hospital bone density can be measured. This helps the patient to know whether the bone is normal or at risk of fracture. Densitometry is the way by which bone density is measured. The diagnoses can be done by using digital xray radiogrammetry, dual photon absorptiometry, single photon absorptiometry, quantitative computed tomography,

quantitative ultrasound, single

energy xray absorptiometry,

dual-energy xray

absorptiometry and dual xray

absorptiometry and laser. This

can be done in the hospital.

The Effects Of Smoking On The Bone:

Smoking of cigarette is not good for the bone health. It result to negative effects to the bones of the body. Vitamin D will not function properly in the absorption of calcium in the bone. This will result to low bone health. It will cause malnourishment of the bones of the body. Smoking reduce the bone density. This makes the bone to be weak. This can result to the bone to be easily fractured. It causes negative effects on the collagen formation. Estrogen is an hormone that is needed to make calcium, magnesium and phosphorus to be retained in the bone. Smoking makes estrogen to be reduced. This makes the minerals to be reduced from the bone. This is demineralization. This therefore makes the bone density to be reduced. This therefore can lead to fracture of the bone. It is also good to be far from areas where there is smoke. Inhaling the smoke has adverse effects on the bone of the body.

Bone Mineral Density:

Bone health can be known by

the use of bone mineral density.

When the bone mineral density

is high it indicate that the bone

is strong and healthy. In this

case, the bone is highly

mineralized. But when the bone

mineral density is low it means

the bone is weak and can easily

fracture.

Fracture Prevention:

Fracture can be prevented by:

1. Doing regular exercise.

Regular exercise increases the

bone density. This makes the

bone to be strong and

osteoporosis is prevented.

Therefore, the bone is not at risk to fracture.

2. It is good for the body to have sunshine in the morning. This makes vitamin D production absorb calcium. This increase bone density. This makes the bone to be strong and healthy. Thereby preventing fracture of the bone.

3. Having a lot of calcium, phosphorus and magnesium from the diet is good. For example, fruits such as lettuce has magnesium, calcium and phosphorus. Milk and cheese has calcium. Also black eyed peas,

broccoli,

cucumber,

turnip,

collard greens and Chinese

cabbage has calcium. Pumpkins

has calcium, magnesium and

phosphorus. Squash has

magnesium and phosphorus.

Kiwi fruits has magnesium,

calcium and phosphorus.

Raspberry has calcium,

magnesium and phosphorus.

Sardines and Salmon has

vitamin D. This helps the bone

to absorb calcium. Also include

magnesium in your diet.

Magnesium is mineral that is

stored in the bone. Food that

has magnesium are: nuts, green

leafy vegetables,

whole grains,

legumes, avocados,

potatoes and also bananas. This

makes the bone to be strong

and healthy. Risk of fracture

that can occur due to weak

bone formation is prevented. It is good to eat food that has high level of vitamin B. Osteoblasts bone cells are produced when the body has a lot of vitamin B12. This makes new bone to be formed. This makes the bone density to be high. This makes fracture of the bone to be prevented.

4. It is good to have balance diet. This makes the body to be

healthy including the bone. The carbohydrates, protein, vitamins, minerals, vegetable oil and water taken as food makes the bone to be strong. This prevent bone diseases. This makes the bone not to be weak. This therefore prevent fracture.

5. Wearing of sit belt in the car is good. Whether driving or not driving. Provided you are in the car, it is good you wear sit belt.

This helps to prevent fracture. It helps to keep the body in a position and not making the body to move out of the car when there is very high break or accident. It is good to use the sit belt and to drive by looking at the traffic light, side mirror and the road very well during driving in order to prevent accident.

6. It is good to have good sleep and rest. This helps in the proper formation of the bone. Growth hormone is produced at night, this helps in the increase of the bone density, thereby preventing fracture of the bone.

Bone Diseases:

1. Osteoporosis: This is when the bone is very weak. There is porosity of the bone. This can occur as a result of too low estrogen level in the body. This can also occur as a result of malnutrition. When food that are beneficial for the formation of bone is very low in consumption it can lead to osteoporosis. It is then good to eat food that can cause

mineralization of the bone. This can help in the building of strong bone. Osteoporosis may occur to women after menopause. It may be as a result of low estrogen. Estrogen is an hormone that helps the bone to retain calcium. Women after menopause are expected to eat more of fruits and vegetables, because this helps in the building up of strong bones. It is also good to eat fish, beans and beef because they are protein food. This helps in the development of the bone.

2. Ostalgia: This is pain that occur to the bone. This can happen after a big hit on the thigh, arms or other parts of the body where there is bone. It can also occur as a result of infection to the bone by virus or bacteria. Bone pain can also

occur due to less sleep. It is good to sleep well so that the body can be refreshed.

3. Osteocarcinoma: This is cancer of the bone. This can occur as a result of mutation of the DNA of the bone cells. This can occur as a result of carcinogenic substances. What can cause cancer are carcinogenic substances. These are UV1 and UV2 ultraviolet

rays from the sun. During the

hot sun period it is good to have

cover from the rays by staying

inside building, use umbrella

and not stay standing out side

under the sun rays.

Refined food can cause cancer.

Synthetic food can cause cancer.

Canned food can cause cancer.

Food that has preservatives in it

can cause cancer. Food that has

additives and colorants can

cause cancer.

It is therefore very good to eat

natural food without additives

and colorants. This can help to

prevent cancer of the bone.

4. Osteonecrosis: This simply

means bone death. This can

occur as a result of

disconnection of the blood

supply to the bone. This can

occur after a fatal accident. It is good to use the sit belt when somebody is in the car. It is also good to use the traffic light and side mirrors when driving to prevent this from happening.

5. Osteitis: This is inflammation of the bone. This can occur after the infection of the bone by pathogens. This can occur after drinking dirty water, not well cooked food, low oral hygiene,

low environmental sanitation,
when the house is dirty, when
not taking of bath and also
when infected from somebody
that is already infected by
communicable disease.

Inflammation of the bone can
also occur after trauma(injury)
to the bone. In inflammation
there is swelling, heat, redness
and pain.

6. Osteoarthritis: This means inflammation of the bone joint. This can occur due to infection by pathogens. This can occur after accident. This may also occur due to malnutrition. Soy food is good for the joints to function properly. Avocado fruit is also good to be eaten for the joint to function properly. It is also good to drink enough of water and eat balanced diet.

Spices are good as antibiotics against pathogens.

7. Osteoarthropathy: This means disease to the bone joint. Cancer can cause it. Cancer occur when there is mutation of the DNA. This can be due to viral, bacteria and other microbial infection. This can also occur due to trauma(injury) to the bone joint.

8. Osteochondritis: This means inflammation to where bone is jointed to the cartilage. This can occur after trauma(injury) and also due to infections by disease causing microorganisms.

9. Osteogenesis imperfecta:

This happens when there is defect in the gene. The gene carry the information that is inherited from parents to offspring.

This means formation of the bone is not normal. The fetus in the womb can be affected by this after the mother takes thalidomide. It is good for the mother to eat natural food that is balanced diet. It is good for her to have enough sleep and rest. It is good for her to have exercise like walking in some distance. These will help to prevent this bone disease from occurring.

10. Osteolysis: This means osteoclast cause resorption of bone matrix.

11. Osteopenia: This means low bone cells. There is low bone density. This can occur due to malnutrition, lack of exercise,

pathogens and when there is no good sleep.

12. Osteomalacia: This means the bone is soft. It can result due to vitamin D deficiency. This can occur due to microbial infections, lack of exercise and malnutrition. This can cause bow legs(genu varum).

13. Osteomyelitis: This is the inflammation of the bone or

bone marrow. It can occur due to infection by pathogens.

14. Osteoclasia: This disease occur when after fracture of the bone, there is reabsorption and destruction of the bone. It is good to go to the hospital when there is fracture, so that there can be diagnoses and alignment of the bone.

15. Osteodystrophy: This is abnormal bone development. This can occur due to renal disease(kidney disease).

16. Osteoarthritis: This occur when the ends of joints wear and this causes inflammation of the joints. This can occur due to over use of the joints and lack of rest.

17. Osteopetrosis: This happens when osteoclasts can not resorb bone it makes bone to be hard in the way that is not normal.

18. Osteosclerosis: This is the bone hard in a way that is not normal. This can occur when there is increase in bone formation by osteoblasts and osteocytes. There is low resorption of bone by osteoclasts. It is good to eat

balance diet and not to over eat

those food that has high

content of calcium, phosphorus

and magnesium alone.

19. Ankylosing spondylitis: This

is inflammation of the joints of

the spine.

20. Paget's disease: Paget's

disease of the bone occur as a

result of defect in the

reformation of the new bone

after resorption of the bone in the system. This can make the bone weak and can fracture. It is good to eat food that has a lot of calcium and vitamin D.

Bone Diagnoses:

This can be done by the use of instruments that can scan the bone. For example, X-ray scan, Ultrasound scan, CT scan and MRI scan. These instruments can be used to diagnose fracture of the bone and cancer of the bone.

Bone Therapy (treatment):

This can be done in the hospital by the use of radiotherapy in the case of bone cancer.

Radiotherapy occur by the use

of X-ray to kill the tumour of the

bone. Chemotherapy is also

used for bone cancer and other

bone diseases. This is by the use

of drugs that are prescribed by

the medical doctor.

In the hospital rheumatologist

attend to the joints of patients.

Orthopedic surgeon help in the

fixation of broken bones, in

order for it to be well aligned.

For recovery purpose

rehabilitation specialist attend

to that area. Radiologist helps in

diagnosis by interpreting the

scan. Preventing complications

are done by family doctor. What

causes the disease can be

diagnosed by pathologist. This is

done in the laboratory by the

use light microscope and

electron microscope.

Back pain: This can occur when

there is injury to the back bone.

This may also occur due to lack

of sleep. In the hospital pain

relieving drug may be

prescribed by the doctor. When

somebody laughs pain relieving

substance which is endorphin is

released from the brain. It is

good to sleep well to prevent

back pain. In the case of injury

(trauma) such should be treated

in the hospital.